The Moontime Harmony Journal

A Place to Chart and Keep Track of Your Moontime Needs and Flows

Donna Wolper

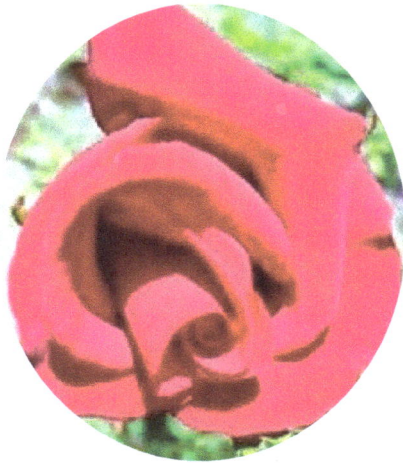

The Moontime Harmony Journal

© 2016 Donna Wolper

ISBN: 978-1-61170-229-3

Cover art by Gina Giommi.

Printed in the USA and UK on acid-free paper.

Rp Robertson Publishing™
www.RobertsonPublishing.com

To purchase additional prints of this book or to purchase
The Moontime Harmony Workbook go to:

amazon.com
barnesandnoble.com

The Moontime Harmony Journal

*T*he Moontime Harmony Journal was created to be used as a helpful *guide* to encourage a spiritual wellness during your menstrual cycle.

It is intended to help a wombyn achieve a love and a deeper understanding of her menstrual cycle or moontime. The intention is to illuminate the blessings of the *Blood Mysteries*, the essence of which has been existing in the dark. The goal is to encourage a wombyn to look forward to her monthly cycle because she will know how to be prepared. A wombyn can learn to listen to the voices of her body, emotions and spirit. This will then help her to build the confidence that she needs to know how to trust her own intuitive intelligence and wisdom. This will help to de-mystify and empower her experience.

It is designed to guide a wombyn for thirteen months, the number of lunar months in a solar year. Each month has a calendar that you can use to chart and follow your rhythms and needs. Each month has a page or two with spaces to journal, answer questions and places to keep track of your physical and emotional needs. These pages offer guidance to a wombyn to help her achieve balance and awareness of her moontime. It points directions and offers reminders so she can follow her moontime experience. It gives her a place to monitor her moontime needs.

It provides spaces to follow your cycles, so you can keep track of what surfaces. This might include keeping an account of what might need to be released or transformed, old negative painful patterns, fears, taboos, or shame. Sources of possible disharmony and pain, once identified, can often be replaced with positive patterns that will unfold a harmonious moontime.

When the lunar light and phases guide a wombyn's experience, moontimes become a spiritual unfolding and an attunement to the Sacred within. Sacred inner worlds emerge, reflecting, like the light of the moon, your own inner Divine energy or connection with the

Goddess. As you align with the *Blood Mysteries*, the essence of the feminine moontime, intuition becomes stronger. Knowing and trusting yourself and your needs becomes clearer. The knowledge of what you require for healing appears and creativity can soar. A wombyn has this opportunity and gift of connection every month. When you do, it's like coming home to yourself.

It is time to transform the disharmonious pain, shame or guilt into the harmonious, sacred, joyous, and illuminated. It is time to love coming home to your own spirit each month. It is time to accept that drifting and dreaming are part of the rhythm and that it will bring you closer to your unconscious, to the void where the Goddess and Divine dwell within. It is time that we honor and rejoice in our inner connection, which is a source of healing and a path to becoming whole. It is time to remember what the *Blood Mysteries* are really about. It is time to reclaim the essence of the Moontime and Divine Feminine because this is your birthright!

HOW TO USE THIS JOURNAL

It has been created to guide a wombyn for 13 months for the purpose of achieving a harmonious moontime.

The journal comes with thirteen calendars, one for each month in a lunar year. Each solar year has thirteen lunar months, each lunar month has twenty eight days. This occurs because the moon takes twenty eight days to wax and wane from one full moon to the next. Menstrual cycles are often twenty eight-day cycles, in harmony with the waxing and waning of the moon. Each month a wombyn waxes and wanes with physical and emotional rhythms in harmony with the moon.

Each calendar is surrounded by a snake. The snake is a symbol of the Goddess energy. A snake sheds its old skin to make room for its new skin. Each month you shed your blood, you not only shed the lining of your uterus, but you also have the opportunity to shed the old and unused parts of yourself and your life to make way for the new. You also have a psychic door that opens to your Goddess space within where you can journey to revisit your Divine inner world. This is what the symbol of the snake represents.

HOW IS THE CALENDAR MEANT TO BE USED?

On the top of the calendar is a place to put the month and the year. Each month has twenty eight days. Each day is divided into twelve boxes for order and convenience. The first two boxes are meant for the number of the day of that month and the lunar phase that that day is in. The remaining ten boxes can be filled in with personal codes for the things you want to follow. They are used to help you keep track and chart your rhythms and *needs of choice* for every day of the month, not just during your moontime.

There is a chart to write down your personal system of coding so you can keep track of the things that you want to follow each month. The situations that you follow can change month to month or stay the same.

You create the code that you want to use for the need that you want to follow. Some choices are to use color, a code letter or a symbol in that will correspond to a particular need. You can also do a combination or come up with your own language of coding that makes sense to you.

For example, cramps. One of the ten boxes can be used to chart your rhythm of cramps by putting a C or the color blue in a box each day that you experience cramping. Many woman have a pattern of cramping and sometimes this pattern can be tracked and even predicted ahead of time. Is that pattern random or predictable? Can you alleviate it if you know ahead of time and perhaps be prepared to take an herb or vitamin that might help? Maybe it is an alert to change your diet a few days before your moontime because you've discovered that certain food choices help minimize or eliminate cramps.

Also included are *thirteen* areas with nine questions and suggestions of things to think about each month. This includes: spaces to journal, a place to write down your dreams, a place for reminders for your needs or path of healing and space to let your creative artistry wander. These questions and spaces are meant to help you keep track of your emotional tides, physical rhythms, patterns, and discoveries. It is a place for keeping track of *moontime* ideas, needs, questions and observations, with spaces to record your personal experiences. These questions are designed to help you get in touch with your unconscious and inner world. The spaces are to be used to record and keep track of the things that you need in order to tend to your physical needs. By tending the garden of your physical needs, you can experience less discomfort. By becoming aware of your psychic life, you can tune into your inner journey. When you *see* or know your *self*, you begin to understand what you may need to include, release, change, create, transform, heal, or just be with each month so that your flow can flow. These situations don't have to be surprises, but can be followed with clarity.

Once you have a format or structure with which to look within, your moontime can be transformed into an experience of comfort, healing and attunement. Your inner home will be comfortably arranged to meet your needs. Instead of there being an unwanted guest each month, you will be the gracious host that invites her home!

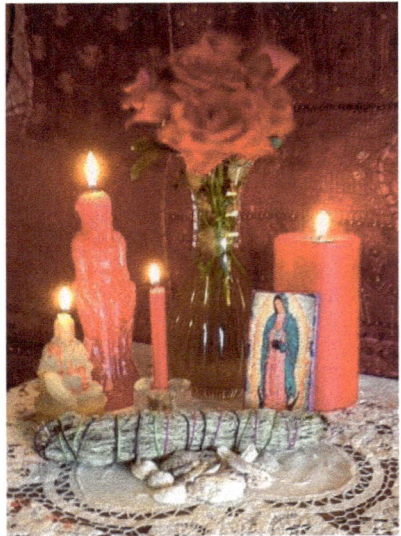

SOME IDEAS for THINGS to CHART and CODE

Bloating	Depression	Days in One's
Cramps	Food Craving	Irritability, Tensions
Acne	Dreaminess	Breast Tenderness
Creativity	Headaches	Changing Sleep
Ovulation	Sexual Changes	Moving In, Out of
Emotional Changes	Vaginal Changes	Desire to be Alone
Moodiness	PMS	Joy

Sleep Patterns-**S,** Cramps-**C**

Depression-**D**

Sexual Changes- **the color scarlet**

Breast Tenderness- **the color violet**

Tensions- **the color brown**

Days in One's Moontime- a **red** or **blue** lunar phase,

Creativity- a rainbow or paint brush,

Food Craving- an ice cream cone

Dreaminess-clouds.

The choices and codes are yours to create, the needs are yours to follow.

Keep track of your own personal moontime codes here, write them down and know you can change or add to them anytime you need too.

Record your personal moontime codes in the following space.

Symbol or Code	What This Symbol or Code Represents
1.	
2.	
3.	
4.	
5.	
6.	
7.	
8.	
9.	
10.	
11.	
12.	
13.	

Here is an example of what one coded day might look like.

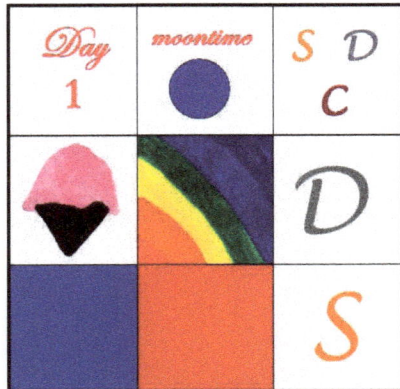

Here is an example of what one week might look like. You can use any combination of coding that inspires you. Create your own codes, place them in a box in each of the week, for each week, for the entire month. After a few months you may see a pattern. When you see this pattern, you can begin to become aware of your rhythms. When you become aware of your rhythms, you can prepare for your needs. When you are prepared, you are in control of the situations instead of them controlling you!

Remember to include the month and year for each calendar.

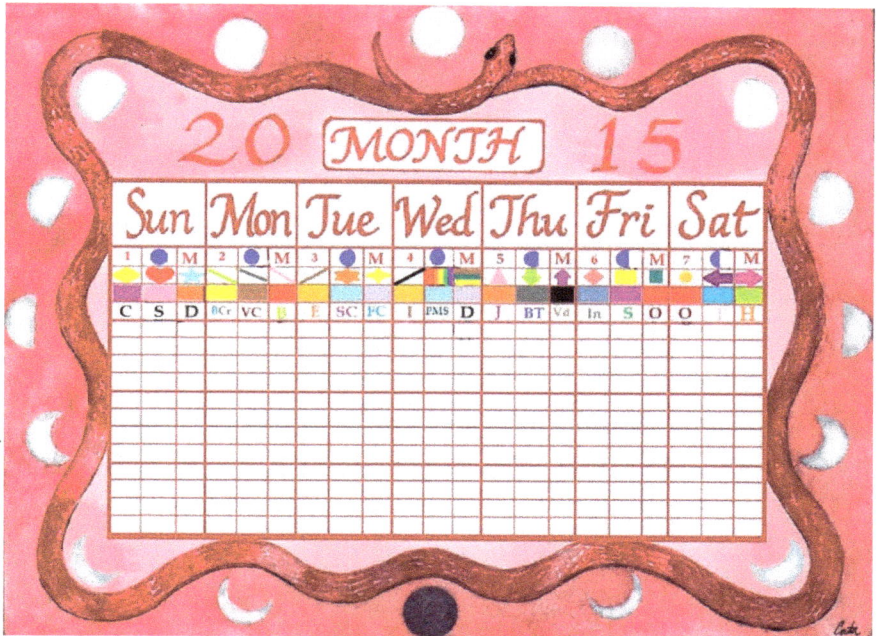

Let's get started!

Sun	Mon	Tue	Wed	Thu	Fri	Sat											

KEEP TRACK OF YOUR FEELINGS AND THOUGHTS HERE

*A*fter the calendar, there are nine places where you can write your personal responses and ideas. The goal is to bring your inner world into the outer world so you can keep track of what is happening to your mind, body, emotions and spirit.

1. Journal - uncensored thoughts, feelings, reactions to this month's moontime.

_____

_____

_____

2. Dreams and Visions - messages from the unconscious, from your Goddess self.

_____

_____

_____

3. Special self-nurturing reminders - things to do for yourself during your moontime, or during the month, to sustain healing.

_____

_____

_____

4. Preparations needed to create a harmonious moontime - reminders for child care, appointments to make or cancel, items to purchase, candles to have for a bath.

_____

_____

_____

_____

5. Reminders for food and diet - when to change or eliminate certain foods, take supplements, herbs to have on hand, things to do that release stress.

_____

_____

_____

6. What old beliefs have been uncovered, need to be eliminated or changed? Create affirmations for transformation.

_____

_____

_____

_____

7. Reminders of activities that will create a harmonious moontime - make an appointment for a massage, walk in nature, get extra sleep, listen to music that you love.

_____

_____

_____

_____

8. What did your last moontime reveal that will help make the next one more spiritual or bring you closer to your sacred self?

_____

_____

_____

_____

9. Create your own ritual, draw or paint your feelings or dreams.

_____

_____

_____

_____

Use These Pages for Notes and Play

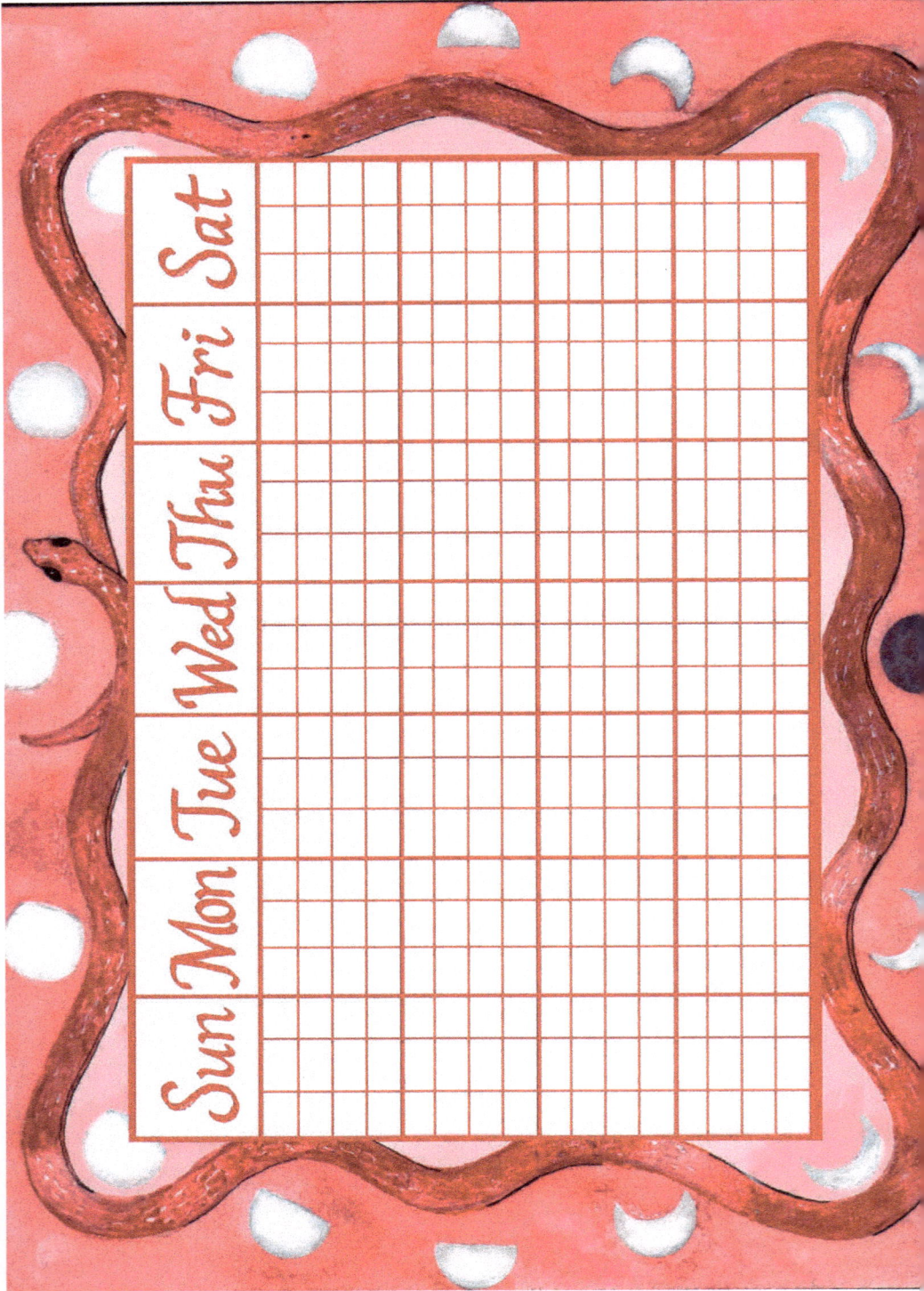

Sun	Mon	Tue	Wed	Thu	Fri	Sat

KEEP TRACK OF YOUR FEELINGS AND THOUGHTS HERE

1. Journal - uncensored thoughts, feelings, reactions to this month's moontime.

_____

_____

_____

_____

2. Dreams and Visions - messages from the unconscious, from your Goddess self.

_____

_____

_____

_____

3. Special self-nurturing reminders - things to do for yourself during your moontime, or during the month, to sustain healing.

_____

_____

_____

_____

4. Preparations needed to create a harmonious moontime - reminders for child care, appointments to make or cancel, items to purchase, candles to have for a bath.

_____

_____

_____

_____

_____

5. Reminders for food and diet - when to change or eliminate certain foods, take supplements, herbs to have on hand, things to do that release stress.

_____

_____

_____

_____

6. What old beliefs have been uncovered, need to be eliminated or changed? Create affirmations for transformation.

_____

_____

_____

_____

7. Reminders of activities that will create a harmonious moontime - make an appointment for a massage, walk in nature, get extra sleep, listen to music that you love.

_____

_____

_____

_____

8. What did your last moontime reveal that will help make the next one more spiritual or bring you closer to your sacred self?

_____

_____

_____

_____

9. Create your own ritual, draw or paint your feelings or dreams.

_____

_____

_____

Use These Pages for Notes and Play

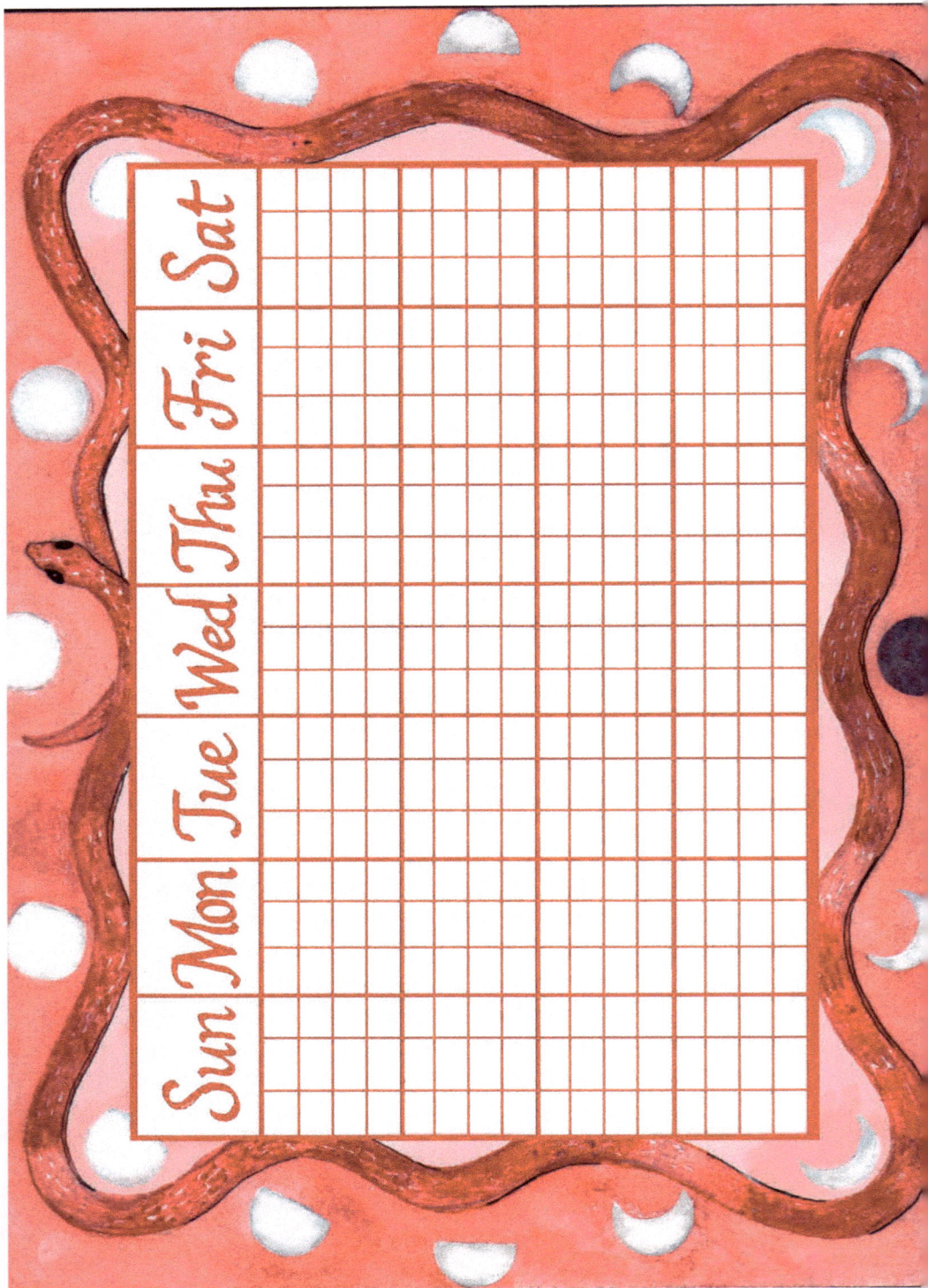

Sun	Mon	Tue	Wed	Thu	Fri	Sat

KEEP TRACK OF YOUR FEELINGS AND THOUGHTS HERE

1. Journal - uncensored thoughts, feelings, reactions to this month's moontime.

_____

_____

_____

_____

2. Dreams and Visions - messages from the unconscious, from your Goddess self.

_____

_____

_____

_____

3. Special self-nurturing reminders - things to do for yourself during your moontime, or during the month, to sustain healing.

_____

_____

_____

_____

4. Preparations needed to create a harmonious moontime - reminders for child care, appointments to make or cancel, items to purchase, candles to have for a bath.

_____

_____

_____

_____

_____

5. Reminders for food and diet - when to change or eliminate certain foods, take supplements, herbs to have on hand, things to do that release stress.

_____

_____

_____

_____

6. What old beliefs have been uncovered, need to be eliminated or changed? Create affirmations for transformation.

_____

_____

_____

_____

7. Reminders of activities that will create a harmonious moontime - make an appointment for a massage, walk in nature, get extra sleep, listen to music that you love.

_____

_____

_____

_____

8. What did your last moontime reveal that will help make the next one more spiritual or bring you closer to your sacred self?

_____

_____

_____

_____

9. Create your own ritual, draw or paint your feelings or dreams.

_____

_____

_____

Use These Pages for Notes and Play

Sun	Mon	Tue	Wed	Thu	Fri	Sat

KEEP TRACK OF YOUR FEELINGS AND THOUGHTS HERE

1. Journal - uncensored thoughts, feelings, reactions to this month's moontime.

_____

_____

_____

_____

2. Dreams and Visions - messages from the unconscious, from your Goddess self.

_____

_____

_____

_____

3. Special self-nurturing reminders - things to do for yourself during your moontime, or during the month, to sustain healing.

_____

_____

_____

_____

4. Preparations needed to create a harmonious moontime - reminders for child care, appointments to make or cancel, items to purchase, candles to have for a bath.

_____

_____

_____

_____

_____

5. Reminders for food and diet - when to change or eliminate certain foods, take supplements, herbs to have on hand, things to do that release stress.

_____
_____
_____
_____

6. What old beliefs have been uncovered, need to be eliminated or changed? Create affirmations for transformation.

_____
_____
_____
_____

7. Reminders of activities that will create a harmonious moontime - make an appointment for a massage, walk in nature, get extra sleep, listen to music that you love.

_____
_____
_____
_____

8. What did your last moontime reveal that will help make the next one more spiritual or bring you closer to your sacred self?

_____
_____
_____
_____

9. Create your own ritual, draw or paint your feelings or dreams.

_____
_____
_____

Use These Pages for Notes and Play

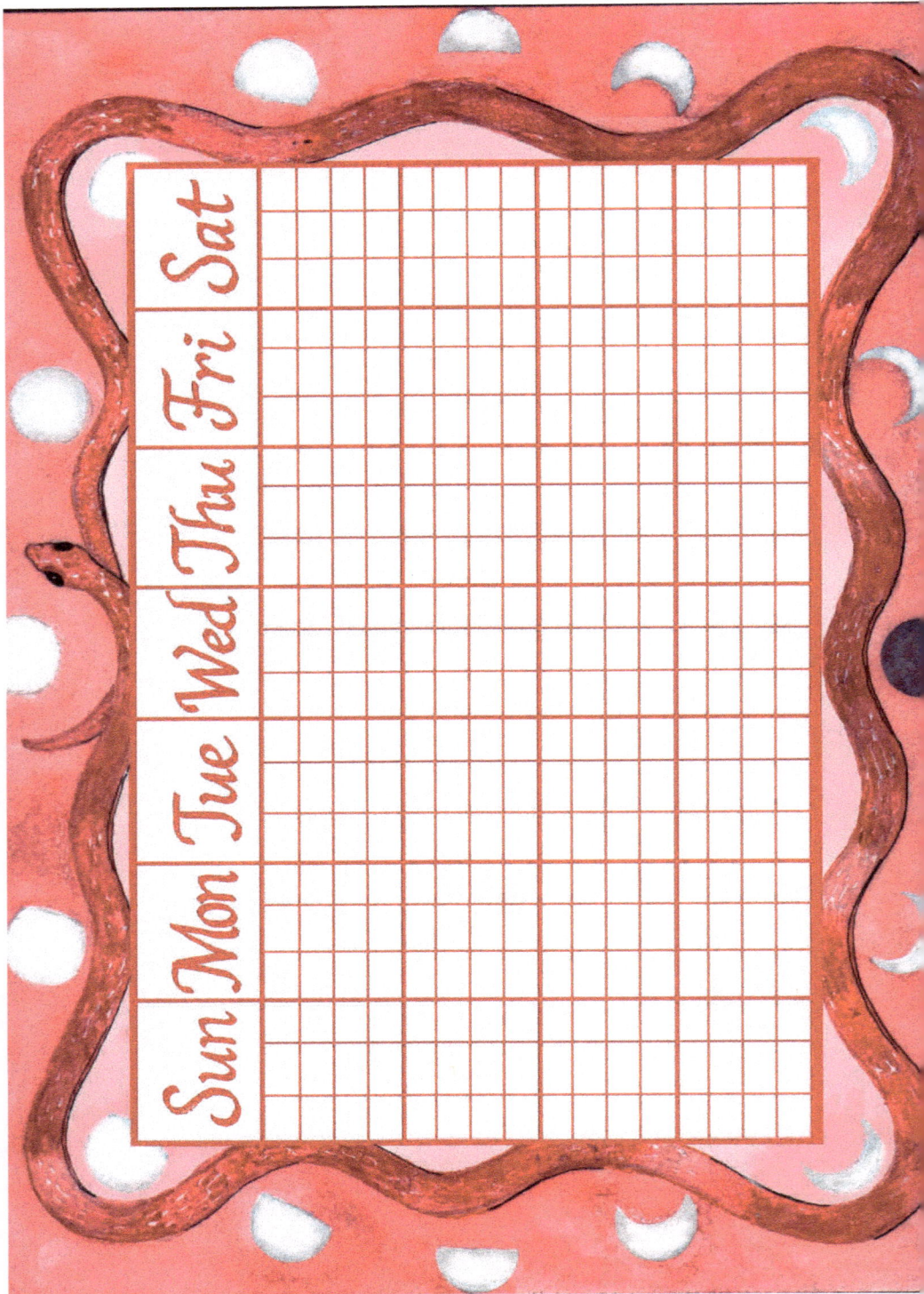

Sun	Mon	Tue	Wed	Thu	Fri	Sat

KEEP TRACK OF YOUR FEELINGS AND THOUGHTS HERE

1. Journal - uncensored thoughts, feelings, reactions to this month's moontime.

_____

_____

_____

_____

2. Dreams and Visions - messages from the unconscious, from your Goddess self.

_____

_____

_____

_____

3. Special self-nurturing reminders - things to do for yourself during your moontime, or during the month, to sustain healing.

_____

_____

_____

_____

4. Preparations needed to create a harmonious moontime - reminders for child care, appointments to make or cancel, items to purchase, candles to have for a bath.

_____

_____

_____

_____

_____

5. Reminders for food and diet - when to change or eliminate certain foods, take supplements, herbs to have on hand, things to do that release stress.

_____

_____

_____

_____

6. What old beliefs have been uncovered, need to be eliminated or changed? Create affirmations for transformation.

_____

_____

_____

_____

7. Reminders of activities that will create a harmonious moontime - make an appointment for a massage, walk in nature, get extra sleep, listen to music that you love.

_____

_____

_____

_____

8. What did your last moontime reveal that will help make the next one more spiritual or bring you closer to your sacred self?

_____

_____

_____

_____

9. Create your own ritual, draw or paint your feelings or dreams.

_____

_____

_____

Use These Pages for Notes and Play

Sun	Mon	Tue	Wed	Thu	Fri	Sat

KEEP TRACK OF YOUR FEELINGS AND THOUGHTS HERE

1. Journal - uncensored thoughts, feelings, reactions to this month's moontime.

_____

_____

_____

_____

2. Dreams and Visions - messages from the unconscious, from your Goddess self.

_____

_____

_____

_____

3. Special self-nurturing reminders - things to do for yourself during your moontime, or during the month, to sustain healing.

_____

_____

_____

_____

4. Preparations needed to create a harmonious moontime - reminders for child care, appointments to make or cancel, items to purchase, candles to have for a bath.

_____

_____

_____

_____

_____

5. Reminders for food and diet - when to change or eliminate certain foods, take supplements, herbs to have on hand, things to do that release stress.

_____

_____

_____

_____

6. What old beliefs have been uncovered, need to be eliminated or changed? Create affirmations for transformation.

_____

_____

_____

_____

7. Reminders of activities that will create a harmonious moontime - make an appointment for a massage, walk in nature, get extra sleep, listen to music that you love.

_____

_____

_____

_____

8. What did your last moontime reveal that will help make the next one more spiritual or bring you closer to your sacred self?

_____

_____

_____

_____

9. Create your own ritual, draw or paint your feelings or dreams.

_____

_____

_____

Use These Pages for Notes and Play

Sun	Mon	Tue	Wed	Thu	Fri	Sat

KEEP TRACK OF YOUR FEELINGS AND THOUGHTS HERE

1. Journal - uncensored thoughts, feelings, reactions to this month's moontime.

_____

_____

_____

_____

2. Dreams and Visions - messages from the unconscious, from your Goddess self.

_____

_____

_____

_____

3. Special self-nurturing reminders - things to do for yourself during your moontime, or during the month, to sustain healing.

_____

_____

_____

_____

4. Preparations needed to create a harmonious moontime - reminders for child care, appointments to make or cancel, items to purchase, candles to have for a bath.

_____

_____

_____

_____

_____

5. Reminders for food and diet - when to change or eliminate certain foods, take supplements, herbs to have on hand, things to do that release stress.

_____

_____

_____

_____

6. What old beliefs have been uncovered, need to be eliminated or changed? Create affirmations for transformation.

_____

_____

_____

_____

7. Reminders of activities that will create a harmonious moontime - make an appointment for a massage, walk in nature, get extra sleep, listen to music that you love.

_____

_____

_____

_____

8. What did your last moontime reveal that will help make the next one more spiritual or bring you closer to your sacred self?

_____

_____

_____

_____

9. Create your own ritual, draw or paint your feelings or dreams.

_____

_____

_____

Use These Pages for Notes and Play

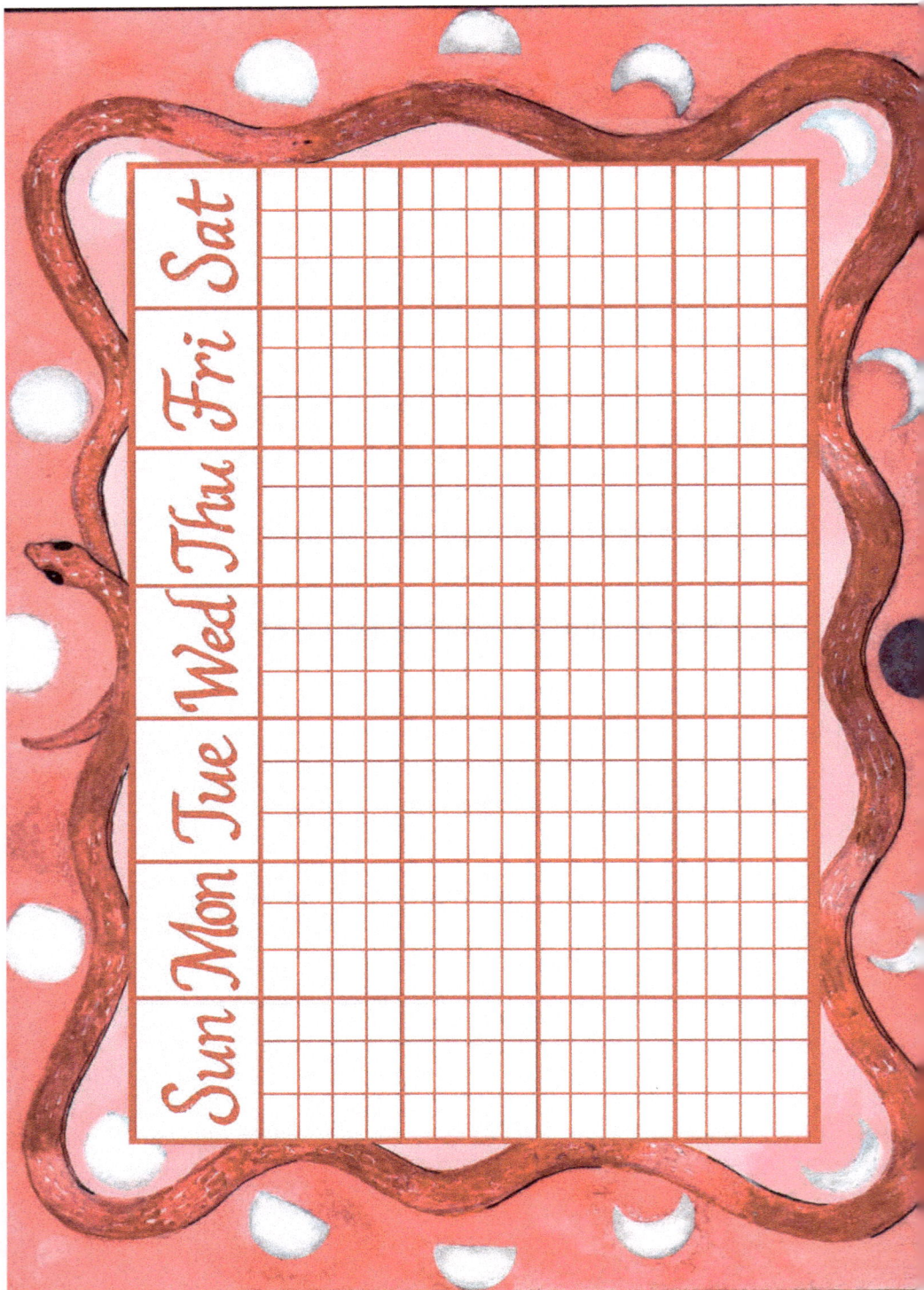

Sun	Mon	Tue	Wed	Thu	Fri	Sat

KEEP TRACK OF YOUR FEELINGS AND THOUGHTS HERE

1. Journal - uncensored thoughts, feelings, reactions to this month's moontime.

_____

_____

_____

_____

2. Dreams and Visions - messages from the unconscious, from your Goddess self.

_____

_____

_____

_____

3. Special self-nurturing reminders - things to do for yourself during your moontime, or during the month, to sustain healing.

_____

_____

_____

_____

4. Preparations needed to create a harmonious moontime - reminders for child care, appointments to make or cancel, items to purchase, candles to have for a bath.

_____

_____

_____

_____

_____

5. Reminders for food and diet - when to change or eliminate certain foods, take supplements, herbs to have on hand, things to do that release stress.

_____
_____
_____
_____

6. What old beliefs have been uncovered, need to be eliminated or changed? Create affirmations for transformation.

_____
_____
_____
_____

7. Reminders of activities that will create a harmonious moontime - make an appointment for a massage, walk in nature, get extra sleep, listen to music that you love.

_____
_____
_____
_____

8. What did your last moontime reveal that will help make the next one more spiritual or bring you closer to your sacred self?

_____
_____
_____
_____

9. Create your own ritual, draw or paint your feelings or dreams.

_____
_____
_____

Use These Pages for Notes and Play

Sun	Mon	Tue	Wed	Thu	Fri	Sat

KEEP TRACK OF YOUR FEELINGS AND THOUGHTS HERE

1. Journal - uncensored thoughts, feelings, reactions to this month's moontime.

_____
_____
_____
_____

2. Dreams and Visions - messages from the unconscious, from your Goddess self.

_____
_____
_____
_____

3. Special self-nurturing reminders - things to do for yourself during your moontime, or during the month, to sustain healing.

_____
_____
_____
_____

4. Preparations needed to create a harmonious moontime - reminders for child care, appointments to make or cancel, items to purchase, candles to have for a bath.

_____
_____
_____
_____
_____

5. Reminders for food and diet - when to change or eliminate certain foods, take supplements, herbs to have on hand, things to do that release stress.

_____

_____

_____

_____

6. What old beliefs have been uncovered, need to be eliminated or changed? Create affirmations for transformation.

_____

_____

_____

_____

7. Reminders of activities that will create a harmonious moontime - make an appointment for a massage, walk in nature, get extra sleep, listen to music that you love.

_____

_____

_____

_____

8. What did your last moontime reveal that will help make the next one more spiritual or bring you closer to your sacred self?

_____

_____

_____

_____

9. Create your own ritual, draw or paint your feelings or dreams.

_____

_____

_____

Use These Pages for Notes and Play

Sun	Mon	Tue	Wed	Thu	Fri	Sat

KEEP TRACK OF YOUR FEELINGS AND THOUGHTS HERE

1. Journal - uncensored thoughts, feelings, reactions to this month's moontime.

_____

_____

_____

_____

2. Dreams and Visions - messages from the unconscious, from your Goddess self.

_____

_____

_____

_____

3. Special self-nurturing reminders - things to do for yourself during your moontime, or during the month, to sustain healing.

_____

_____

_____

_____

4. Preparations needed to create a harmonious moontime - reminders for child care, appointments to make or cancel, items to purchase, candles to have for a bath.

_____

_____

_____

_____

_____

5. Reminders for food and diet - when to change or eliminate certain foods, take supplements, herbs to have on hand, things to do that release stress.

_____

_____

_____

_____

6. What old beliefs have been uncovered, need to be eliminated or changed? Create affirmations for transformation.

_____

_____

_____

_____

7. Reminders of activities that will create a harmonious moontime - make an appointment for a massage, walk in nature, get extra sleep, listen to music that you love.

_____

_____

_____

_____

8. What did your last moontime reveal that will help make the next one more spiritual or bring you closer to your sacred self?

_____

_____

_____

_____

9. Create your own ritual, draw or paint your feelings or dreams.

_____

_____

_____

Use These Pages for Notes and Play

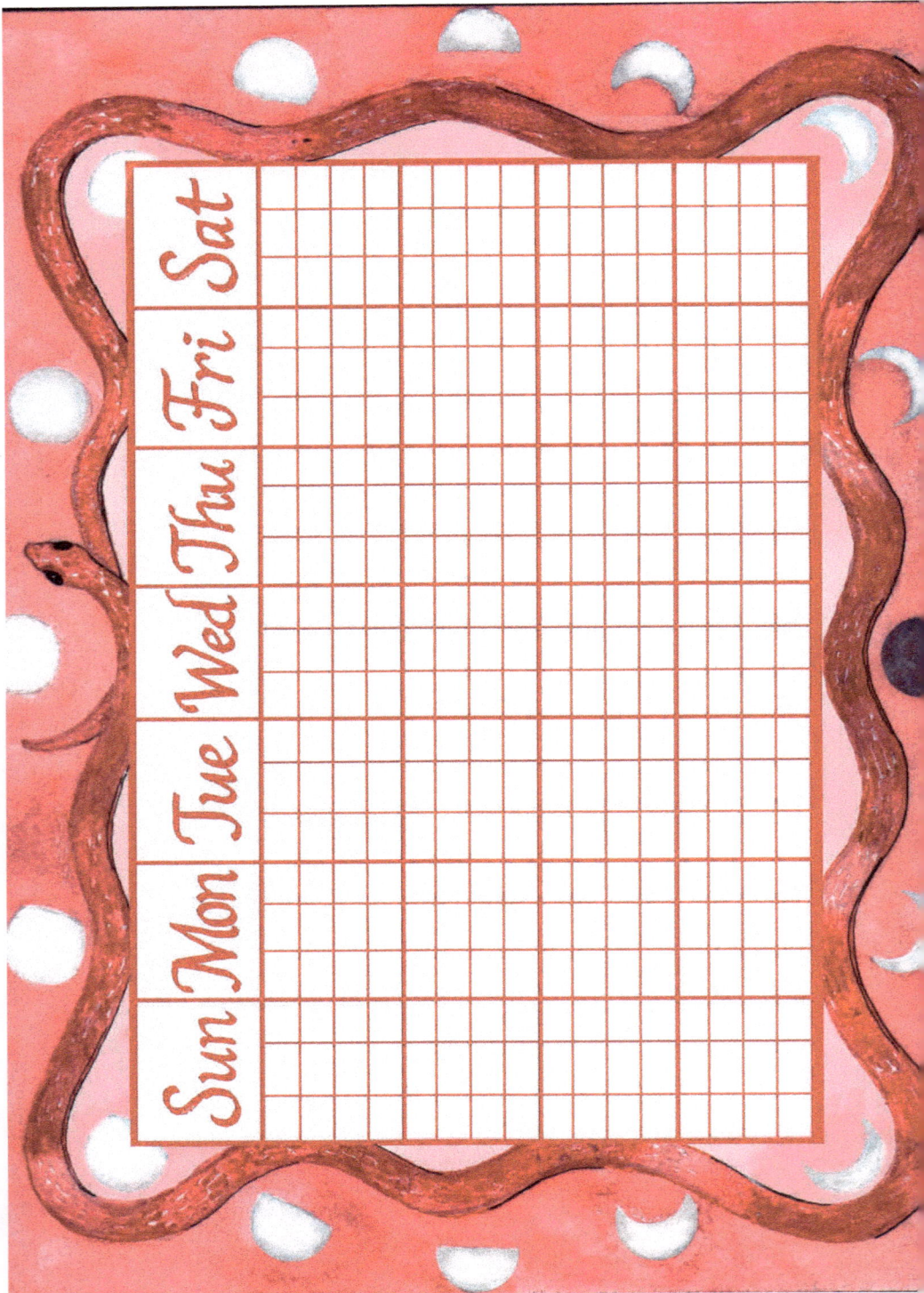

KEEP TRACK OF YOUR FEELINGS AND THOUGHTS HERE

1. Journal - uncensored thoughts, feelings, reactions to this month's moontime.

_____
_____
_____
_____

2. Dreams and Visions - messages from the unconscious, from your Goddess self.

_____
_____
_____
_____

3. Special self-nurturing reminders - things to do for yourself during your moontime, or during the month, to sustain healing.

_____
_____
_____
_____

4. Preparations needed to create a harmonious moontime - reminders for child care, appointments to make or cancel, items to purchase, candles to have for a bath.

_____
_____
_____
_____
_____

5. Reminders for food and diet - when to change or eliminate certain foods, take supplements, herbs to have on hand, things to do that release stress.

_____

_____

_____

_____

6. What old beliefs have been uncovered, need to be eliminated or changed? Create affirmations for transformation.

_____

_____

_____

_____

7. Reminders of activities that will create a harmonious moontime - make an appointment for a massage, walk in nature, get extra sleep, listen to music that you love.

_____

_____

_____

_____

8. What did your last moontime reveal that will help make the next one more spiritual or bring you closer to your sacred self?

_____

_____

_____

_____

9. Create your own ritual, draw or paint your feelings or dreams.

_____

_____

_____

Use These Pages for Notes and Play

Sun	Mon	Tue	Wed	Thu	Fri	Sat

KEEP TRACK OF YOUR FEELINGS AND THOUGHTS HERE

1. Journal - uncensored thoughts, feelings, reactions to this month's moontime.

_____

_____

_____

_____

2. Dreams and Visions - messages from the unconscious, from your Goddess self.

_____

_____

_____

_____

3. Special self-nurturing reminders - things to do for yourself during your moontime, or during the month, to sustain healing.

_____

_____

_____

_____

4. Preparations needed to create a harmonious moontime - reminders for child care, appointments to make or cancel, items to purchase, candles to have for a bath.

_____

_____

_____

_____

_____

5. Reminders for food and diet - when to change or eliminate certain foods, take supplements, herbs to have on hand, things to do that release stress.

_____

_____

_____

_____

6. What old beliefs have been uncovered, need to be eliminated or changed? Create affirmations for transformation.

_____

_____

_____

_____

7. Reminders of activities that will create a harmonious moontime - make an appointment for a massage, walk in nature, get extra sleep, listen to music that you love.

_____

_____

_____

_____

8. What did your last moontime reveal that will help make the next one more spiritual or bring you closer to your sacred self?

_____

_____

_____

_____

9. Create your own ritual, draw or paint your feelings or dreams.

_____

_____

_____

Use These Pages for Notes and Play

Sun	Mon	Tue	Wed	Thu	Fri	Sat

KEEP TRACK OF YOUR FEELINGS AND THOUGHTS HERE

1. Journal - uncensored thoughts, feelings, reactions to this month's moontime.

_____

_____

_____

_____

2. Dreams and Visions - messages from the unconscious, from your Goddess self.

_____

_____

_____

_____

3. Special self-nurturing reminders - things to do for yourself during your moontime, or during the month, to sustain healing.

_____

_____

_____

_____

4. Preparations needed to create a harmonious moontime - reminders for child care, appointments to make or cancel, items to purchase, candles to have for a bath.

_____

_____

_____

_____

_____

5. Reminders for food and diet - when to change or eliminate certain foods, take supplements, herbs to have on hand, things to do that release stress.

_____
_____
_____
_____

6. What old beliefs have been uncovered, need to be eliminated or changed? Create affirmations for transformation.

_____
_____
_____
_____

7. Reminders of activities that will create a harmonious moontime - make an appointment for a massage, walk in nature, get extra sleep, listen to music that you love.

_____
_____
_____
_____

8. What did your last moontime reveal that will help make the next one more spiritual or bring you closer to your sacred self?

_____
_____
_____
_____

9. Create your own ritual, draw or paint your feelings or dreams.

_____
_____
_____

Use These Pages for Notes and Play

Use These Pages for Notes and Play

Use These Pages for Notes and Play

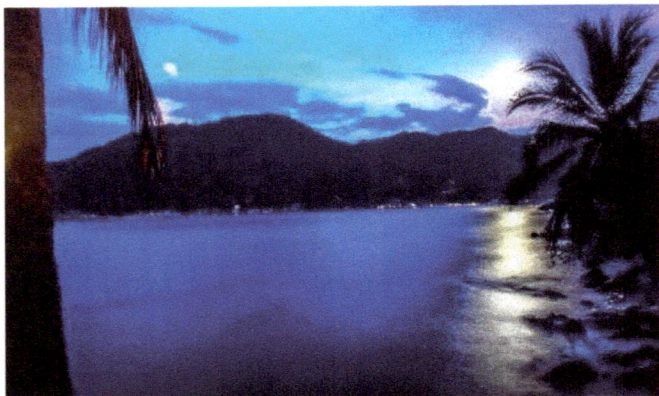

$\mathcal{I}$ spent many years living in a coastal, jungle, fishing village in Mexico. In those early days, the village did not have any electricity, cars or roads. Even today the village still exists without cars and roads, while the main access is by boat.

I lived there for many years, sometimes with my children, sometimes without. Usually I stayed at least 6 months and each time I began to attune to the harmonies and rhythms of the moon, tides and the natural world. It was through this attunement that my menstrual cycle-my moontime- aligned with the phases of the moon and the information for this book surfaced.

Each year that I returned, more clarity emerged and the rhythms of the *Blood Mysteries* deepened. I finally became aware of my phases and cycles and their interconnectedness with the moon and nature. I embraced this physical part of myself, while opening up to the Divine within. I became familiar with the signposts that helped me navigate my way into the inner garden of the Goddess and began listening to Her messages. I recognized patterns that could be healed, alignments with the phases of the moon, rhythms that could be charted and followed. Each month I began to come home to myself and realized that if I could, any wombyn could. It became clear that once a wombyn knew and understood how to take these conscious steps, she could connect with this Goddess given gift.

I began to keep track of my physical and emotional changes each month. Once in my moontime, I could let go and travel into my inner world where the veil lifted and the Sacred was revealed. I observed that if I honored that flow, I emerged renewed, felt whole and moved out into the world with more joy, ease and energy. Thus the idea for a book—a format to keep track, observe, monitor and follow my needs and rhythmic changes—was born. Once the book was finished, this journal became my next focus.

This is the process that I want to share with every *wombyn** in the hope that I can offer a way to understand and demystify your own moontime cycle. It is by illuminating the knowledge of the patterns of your rhythms, that you can embrace your moontime with the awareness that the Goddess intended.

You'll notice I prefer the spelling of *wombyn** instead of *woman* and use the spelling *wembyn** to denote the plural. I believe that the source of our feminine harmony is connected to our wombs; this spelling helps me to remember that connection.

So may the truth of the *Blood Mysteries* be alive within every *wombyn* and may this balance ripple out into the entire world.

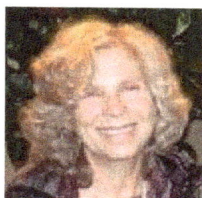

Donna Wolper
Sept. 30, 2015
Santa Cruz, CA. 95060
www.moontimeharmony.com
moontimeharmony@gmail.com
Daily Om course Healing Your
Menstrual Moontime www.dailyom.com

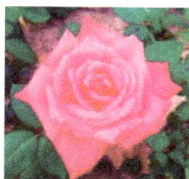

Thank you to Gina Giommi for her expert and beautiful journal cover and help with the calendar. The most super nifty of wonderful people!

www.ingramcontent.com/pod-product-compliance
Lightning Source LLC
Chambersburg PA
CBHW051432270326
41934CB00018B/3482